PMS CURE

Easy To Follow Home Remedies For PMS & PMDD

Introduction

<u>Don't let menstrual cramps make your life miserable when you can use readily available natural remedies to ease the pain and discomfort!</u>

<u>**Do you always have to deal with menstrual cramps each time you have your period**? Are you tired of twisting and turning in your bed or chair just trying to find the best position that will reduce the pain? Have you ended up relying too much on drugs such that you are just helpless without the drugs? Are **you looking for an easy way to manage the pain and be free to engage in daily activities even when on your period?**</u>

If you are, then you have to love this book.

This short, simple to follow book was specifically created for you to help you with dealing with pain.

My wife has been there and seeing the pain she has had to go through just prompted me to do what I do best i.e. research for the best solutions for easing the pain. And after months of research, she started experimenting with different natural solutions to find what works. I can honestly say that the stuff in here works because I have seen it work for my wife.

<u>This book has various home remedies that my wife has used over the years for managing the pain and have been very effective and I know they will be of great help to you too.</u>

More precisely, in this book, you will learn:

- *What causes menstrual cramps and why it the cramps vary*

- ***The different types of menstrual cramps that you may experience***

- *The different strategies you can use to relieve menstrual pain*

- ***How to use exercises to relieve menstrual pain***

- *How to use heat to relieve menstrual pain*

- ***How to leverage on the power of aromatherapy and abdominal massage to relieve menstrual cramps***

- *How to make use diet to overcome menstrual cramps*

- ***And much, much more!***

If you are desperate to get relief from menstrual cramps, this book is for you.

I hope you enjoy it!

PS: I'd like your feedback. If you are happy with this book, please leave a review on Amazon.

Please leave a review for this book on Amazon by visiting the page below:

https://amzn.to/2VMR5qr

Table of Contents

Menstrual Cramps: What Causes The Pain And Why Does It Vary

Menstrual cramps are sharp pains that you feel in your lower abdomen with your every menstrual period. The medical term given for this pain is **dysmenorrhea.** You may have the cramps at the beginning of your menstrual period or they may even go on for as long as you have your periods. The pain varies with every woman and may range from a mild annoying pain to very severe pains that might distract you from your daily activities. Amazingly, the pain does not happen to all women. However, for others it is a completely different story. The pain is usually too much for some women making them not make it to work. Actually, menstrual cramps have been established to be the leading cause of absenteeism for many women in work.

You are more likely to have menstrual cramps if:

- You started your periods at an early age that is less than 11 years

- Your menstrual periods last for five days or longer

- You have relatives who have them

- You smoke cigarettes

What Causes The Pain?

You may wonder why you have the pain in the first place. The exact cause of the menstrual cramps are not known for a fact. However, there are many explanations for what causes the pain.

The scientific explanation for what causes the pain is that; when the uterine lining that is shed every month begins to break down; your body releases chemicals that are known as prostaglandins. The chemicals cause the uterine muscles to contract. As the muscles contract, the blood vessels to the muscles are also constricted. This limits the blood supply to the muscles and as a result, the oxygen level in the muscles and the tissue reduces. The tissues that lack oxygen then dic and slough off causing the bleeding. Remember that the blood supply is cut to the dying tissues and reduced to the surrounding muscles. The lack of oxygen in these muscles causes the pain.

Why Does The Pain Vary?

It is believed that each woman produces different levels of these chemicals called prostaglandins. If you produce high levels of prostaglandins then your contractions are going to be stronger and your pain more severe.

Types Of Menstrual Pains

Scientifically, the menstrual pains can be classified into two. The classification comes about because of the causes. The two types of menstrual pains are:

Primary; this is mainly seen in young women; those who have just started their menstrual periods. It occurs in the absence of any anatomical abnormalities or underlying medical conditions

Secondary; this occurs mainly due to an underlying medical condition. It occurs among older women between the ages of 30-45. To manage secondary dysmenorrhea (menstrual cramps), you will need medical/pharmacological help because it may be a little advanced. If your painful periods are caused by an underlying medical condition, you will have other symptoms like;

- Irregular periods

- Bleeding or spotting in between your periods

- Foul smelling vaginal discharge

- Feeling pain during sexual intercourse

If you experience a change in your normal period pattern or even the pain then it is important that you see a doctor.

The next chapters will address various home remedies that can help you deal with menstrual cramps.

Exercises To Relieve Menstrual Pain

Exercising does help in reducing menstrual pain. Exercising for three to four days in a week is excellent for your health. Additionally, when you exercise you, release some endorphins, which in turn counteract the effects of prostaglandins hence making you feel relieved. Therefore, exercise is especially helpful during your menstrual periods.

Do Exercises Sometimes Worsen The Pain?

While exercise can help reduce the menstrual pain, they may also worsen the pain at times. However, this only happens when your body has low calcium or magnesium levels. The muscles will tend to tense even more and hence worsen the pain. Nevertheless, I have a solution to this that I have discussed later in the book. You can improve both your calcium and magnesium levels by simply adjusting your diet.

Exercises That Help Relieve Menstrual Cramps

The exercises that help relieve the pains don't have to be vigorous. You can decide to brisk walk or jog if you can. I know this may seem difficult because of the pain. However, it will not hurt to try them. Furthermore, when in pain, you have just got to try everything to address with the pain so you might as well exercise. Below are some exercises that you can engage in:

- Abdominal exercises

You can take a fifteen minutes walk. While you are walking, try to contract and release your abdominal muscles. Aim for at least one strong contraction every minute.

You can also get to a sit up position on the floor, and then clasp your knee to your chest and hold for 10 seconds then relax. Do this ten times.

- Yoga poses

Yoga emphasizes on deep breathing and relaxation exercises that can help you reduce the pain. You can lie on your back and place your legs against the wall. This stretches your back and relieves the pain. You can also simply sit crossing your legs and performing deep breathing exercises. By this I mean you deeply inhale and the slowly exhale. This is also a very relaxing exercise.

- Swimming

Swimming is classified as a low impact exercise that does not cause unnecessary strain on your body. It, however, exercises your heart and makes you release the feel-good hormones helping you relieve the pain. You can do this in warm water to achieve a double effect; both the relieving effects of the exercise and the heat.

- Stretching

Stretching exercises are also good at relieving tension in your muscles and hence relieving the pain. Choose a stretching exercise depending on where the pain is. The stretching exercises can be performed as many times as you can during the day.

For cramps in the back and abdomen, lie on your back with your buttocks as close to the wall as possible. Place your legs against the wall then spread them out as much as you can. Hold them there for as long as possible before you relax

For cramps in your back, sit on a chair then try to reach your ankle, in a way that makes you feel like you are tying the laces of your shoe. Once there, hold on for as long as possible.

Another general but good one is trunk rotation where you lie on your back and extend your arms. Then lift your knee to an upright position and swing it to the right for a minute. After which you can swing it to the left for another minute. This can repeatedly be done until you feel some relief.

- Having an orgasm i.e. have sex or masturbate

Just like exercises, orgasms help to release all kinds of pain. The mechanism leading to this is; before an orgasm, the uterine is very relaxed. This increases the blood flow to the uterine muscles. Since blood has oxygen, its increase helps to relieve the pain. There is also another aspect of orgasms, which is helping you to produce endorphins that make you feel better instantly. After an orgasm, you usually feel relaxed and you may easily fall asleep; this is another way that orgasm provides relief.

Remember, exercises will increase blood flow to your entire body, and this brings oxygen with it. Oxygen, in this case, is your medicine.

Apply Heat

Applying heat on your lower abdomen is one of the easiest ways to relieve menstrual pains. Experts believe that heat helps to relax the uterine muscles that are usually contracting and making you feel the pain. You can use various ways to apply heat on your lower abdomen. One of the modern ways is buying a heating pad. These are available in many forms, use electricity, and are reusable. Other ways can be by use of hot water bottles. These bottles are available in many retail shops. The bottles come in different lovely colors and comfortable cushioning too.

How to do it

Place a heating pad or a hot water bottle over the lower part of your abdomen or your lower back. Keep applying the heat until you feel comfortable. This will take only a few minutes. Alternatively, if a water bottle is not available, get a towel and soak it in cold water. Wring out the excess water then place it in a microwave until it is warm. You can then place this over your lower abdomen and your back until it cools. Always change to another warm one once it cools. You can keep doing this until you feel some relief.

In addition to using the heat pads and hot water bottles, all you may need is just to take a hot shower, and you can get instant relief.

Abdominal and Aromatherapy Massage

The goal of a massage is to reduce pelvic congestion from the hormones rushing to the uterus. There are different types of massages that you can do:

Abdominal massage; You can massage your abdomen for five minutes per day, starting six days before you start having your menstrual periods to the start date. This massage increases uterine circulation and reduces localized muscle tension.

Aromatherapy massage; This is simply a massage with different types of essential oil that may help to reduce the pain. There are specific essential oils known to have a relaxing effect on the mind and also to cramping muscles. Examples of these include lavender oil, rosemary, chamomile, cypress, sage, and ginger. The massage can be done on the abdomen, hips and lower back to reduce the uterine pain.

How to Do the Body Massage on Yourself

1. Find a peaceful and relaxing place.

2. Make a blend of 5ml almond oil, 1 drop rose essential oil, 1 drop clary sage essential oil and 1 drop lavender.

3. Smear the blend onto your palm and gently apply it to your abdomen

4. Slowly move your palm in a clockwise circular motion around your belly button for a minute. The belly button is believed to have sensitive spots that can help reduce the pain if adequate pressure is applied.

5. Widen the circumference of your massage area to the whole abdomen slowly to relieve the pain.

6. Place both of your hands at either side of your belly button with your thumbs close to the fingers almost touching them. Moving your fingers downwards and outwards. Try to draw the shape of a heart moving it back to the original position. Repeat this movement severally.

7. Then place your hands on the back, just below the ribs, then apply some pressure and move down just above your hips. From the center of your back, massage in circular motions and move outwards to the corners of your hips. Slide your hand up and repeat this massage thrice.

While abdominal massage is very effective in addressing menstrual cramps, you should avoid this massage if:

- You suffer from irritable bowel disease or,

- You have been diagnosed to have uterine fibroids

Diet: What to Eat and What to Avoid

As much as there is evidence that the pains are hormonal, management of the pain can focus on areas that produce the hormones rather than handling the hormones themselves. This is where diet comes in, as it may either improve or worsen the symptoms. Experts think that the amount of estrogen that is a primary hormone in our cycle can be reduced by a low-fat diet and a high fiber diet.

It is believed that animal products facilitate estrogen reabsorption and added oil while its reabsorption can be blocked by fiber found in grains, vegetables, beans and other plant foods. In terms of nutrients, the following have been established to reduce the production of prostaglandins and speed up their elimination

Calcium; this is known for relieving muscle tension. It is available in dark leafy vegetables like kales and broccoli, low-fat milk and yogurt.

Magnesium; deficiency of magnesium can worsen menstrual cramps. In order to get magnesium, you can eat cashew nuts, pinto beans, and wheat germ

Vitamin E; May inhibit prostaglandin formation. This vitamin is found in sunflower seed and almonds.

What are the specific foods that you can eat?

Ginger; this spice plays a role in the reduction of prostaglandins. It also helps in the management of fatigue during your periods and has the effect of making your periods regular.

Grate a small piece of ginger, bring it to boil in a pot, add honey or lemon to taste and drink this thrice a day during your periods. You can also cook your food with it.

Basil; this contains caffeic acid that has painkilling properties

Crush a handful of basil leaves to extract the juice. Add two teaspoons of the juice to warm water. Drink this three times a day during your menstrual periods

Cinnamon; this has properties that act against muscle spasms and inflammation hence reducing the pain. It is also rich in dietary fiber, calcium, and iron.

Add one-quarter teaspoon of cinnamon powder in a cup of warm water. Stir it and then add honey or lemon to taste.

Drink two to three cups of cinnamon tea before your period starts.

Fennel; this helps relax the muscles in the uterus

Add one teaspoon of fennel seeds to a cup of boiling water. Simmer the mixture on low heat for five minutes. Add one teaspoon of honey and mix well. Drink the tea (keep it hot for best results) two to three days before your period begins.

Blackstrap Molasses; this is rich in iron, calcium, potassium and magnesium. It also soothes the uterine muscles easing the pain.

Add one to two teaspoons of blackstrap molasses to a cup of warm milk. Drink it as soon as you start having cramps and continue as long as needed.

Papaya; this helpful in treating cramps, and it has anti-inflammatory properties. Papaya is also rich in calcium, iron, carotene, vitamin A, and C.

In addition to considering the specific foods and spices that can contribute to reducing menstrual pains, it is also important to find a general diet that you should follow that will help you manage menstrual cramps. For adequate management of menstrual cramps, your diet then should have plenty of:

#Whole grains; Examples of whole grains are like oatmeal, whole grain, brown rice and whole grain bread.

#Vegetables; Such vegetables include Brussels sprouts, sweet potatoes, carrots, spinach, and broccoli.

#Legumes; these are like lentils, peas and beans

#Fruits

In addition to the above that you should eat, you also need to reduce the intake of certain foods that are known to worsen menstrual cramps.

- Animal products; red meat, and too much of poultry products. It is advisable to eat white meat if you have to take meat. However, ensure that you take a limited amount.

- Added vegetable oils; these are salad dressings and margarine

- Fatty foods; examples of foods that have too much fat are French fries, potato chips, ice cream etc. You should avoid too much peanut butter.

- Sugars; refined sugar triggers an increase in the release of insulin and when too much insulin is produced, more prostaglandins are also released.

- Coffee, Alcohol, Carbonated drinks; caffeine worsens the condition.

Conclusion

We've come to the end of the book. Thank you for reading until the end.

I hope this book was able to help you to know how to manage menstrual cramps without having to rely on medication each time.

The next step is to start by adapting a healthy diet so that you can start preparing yourself to manage the pain before it even starts.

As you are aware, menstrual cramps can make it very hard for you to go on with your daily activities as you should and this can cause great strain on your work and your business simply because you have to take a break whenever you have your menstrual periods. For most people, we turn to drugs. However, my wife tried that for years and she ended up being too dependent on the drugs such that she could not function without the drugs. That was until she started using the natural remedies discussed in this book.

With the home remedies outlined in this book, you need not rely on drugs ever again.

Now is your turn to take action!

PS: I'd like your feedback. If you are happy with this book, please leave a review on Amazon.

Please leave a review for this book on Amazon by visiting the page below:

https://amzn.to/2VMR5qr